WE'RE STILL HEAVY:

A Weight Loss Journey

by

Andrew Jenkins

We're Still Heavy: A Weight Loss Journey Copyright © 2018 by Andrew Jenkins. All Rights Reserved.

All rights reserved. No part of this book may be reproduced in any form or by any electronic or mechanical means including information storage and retrieval systems, without permission in writing from the author. The only exception is by a reviewer, who may quote short excerpts in a review.

Cover designed by Andrew Jenkins

This book is a work of nonfiction. Any resemblance to actual persons, living or dead, events, or locales is entirely coincidental.

Andrew Jenkins
Visit my website at www.AuthorName.com

Printed in the United States of America

First Printing: December 2018
Self-Published at Amazon: Kindle Direct Publishing

ISBN-9781791582814

PREFACE

My name is Andrew. As I write this, approximately 2/5 of Americans are obese, while roughly half are trying to lose weight. I have been overweight my entire life. This book holds everything I have learned on my own weight loss journey for the past 14 years. I wish I knew back then as much as I know now. I have fought against nicotine addiction, and caffeine dependence, as well as food habits just bad enough to leave stretch marks on every one of my limbs. I placed videos on YouTube about various things I've learned, generating more than 40,000+ views on my channel. The thankful comments have inspired me to create more content. It would be a waste if I didn't share my past 14 years of internet research on dieting & Exercise. I want to inform you about various aspects of exercises suited for your size & weight. I will explain important facts on the nutritional label. We'll know the differences between good fats vs bad fats plus the good cholesterol vs the bad cholesterol. We will also understand how to use low to high carbs with low to high calories, allowing us to increase our food options. These things and more come first. However, if you are interested in diet pills, those can be found in the back of this book. I'm not selling pills, so please do not get the wrong idea. You can even buy any brand name you like. Two of the supplements work as an aide against consuming more junk (sweets and fats) plus having smaller portions. If you take the pills, reading this book will add to your success. I stress patience with weight loss. The worst mistake people make is becoming too anxious over fast results. I can't count how many times I stepped on the scale, reading a three pound gain, only to become completely discouraged. Afterwards, I felt like giving up on dieting and exercise altogether. However, while I was away from diet & exercise, I never stopped forever. I kept searching the inter-web for answers. As long as we keep searching for answers to help us achieve our weight loss goals, we will never be considered quitters. What I am saying is that breaks are ok. But, during a break, figure out what went wrong. Keep studying. If we keep looking & apply what we learn, then weight loss is just around the corner.

CONTENTS

USEFUL INFORMATION: 37

PHYSICAL APECTS:

EXERCISE VS DIETING:

In the first quarter of this book we will go over several topics about exercise. There are many people losing weight through exercise. If you can push yourself hard enough to lose weight, then I envy you. The more challenging the workouts become, the harder the weight is on our knees, as well as our heart and lungs.

There is a simple approach to explain why we have so much more trouble getting exercise when we have unnecessary body weight. Visualize pulling a 50 pound ball of flesh from your body. (50pds= almost 6 gallons of milk.) This ball of flesh is skin on the exterior. Inside is fat around muscle filled with veins and arteries.

Plug this 50 pound ball of nerves & arteries into your heart and lungs. The heart must now work twice as hard to pump blood through this 50 pound mass. Additionally, every cell needs oxygen, so your lungs must work harder. Now try jogging with it!

This is why exercise gets so much easier after dropping 50 pounds. Your body will not have to produce so much insulin, and your resting heart rate will go down as well. (There's more about heart rates & diabetes later on.

(ABC) 3 BASIC TYPES OF EXERCISE:

There are three key exercise methods with different outcomes.

a) Produces leaner muscle.

b) Produces larger muscles.

c) Is best for improving endurance. (Heart & Lunges.)

Option a) is low intensity (less resistance) exercise for long periods of time. (There are many repetitions, aka reps) We need to feel a burn. This method creates cuts. The "cut" is a term for working out to become leaner. The body will be appear "cut" aka "chiseled".

Ex. Adjusting a gym bike to a low strength setting for 30-60 minutes is a good example of a low impact/high rep/ workout. Using your lighter free weights with many reps is another example.

Option b) is the use of a safe, high resistance/high weight as much as you can, for only a few reps. Option b is great for building muscle.

One mistake people make with ab workouts is that they use option b). The result is a belly that sticks out from building ab muscle, but no fat loss. I made this mistake myself for many years.

You can use options a) and b) strategically. Use option a) for your legs to trim down. If a guy wants bigger arms, then option b) is preferred.

Option c) is cardio workouts. Cardio greatly improves stamina while burning fat more than the other two options. Cardio can include exercises from a) & b).

Cardio is achieved through any movement raising the heart rate to a high, yet safe, number.

EMBARRASSMENT:

Most people understand how embarrassing workouts can be, especially on walks, going to the gym, and jogging.

Over the years I have learned that getting started is the hardest part of anything difficult. Applying for a job, your first day at school, the first day at work, studying for a test, starting house chores, and walks, can all be difficult at first. Just get started and you will feel better afterwards.

In my 20's, exercise videos on TV were available. I was frozen at the thought of trying out the exercises, even though I was completely alone in my house. I was like a deer caught in the light of my television screen. I literally sweated without moving, thinking that someone would see me looking foolish. Eventually, I took a deep breath, and tried an exercise. It felt good.

An entire 15 minute workout was too much for me, so my best option was to ease my way in. When I saw an ab movement I liked, I tried it out on the floor. After breaking the ice, I kept trying new moves.

I made that first leap 14 years ago, and I am now capable of most individual ab exercises.

Every day adds up to a stronger future. Let's do the math for one entire year. 10 push-ups a day times 365 days= 3,650 push-ups a year. 10 crunches= 3,650 crunches a year. 10 years makes 36,500 of each exercise.

If we can only perform 1 pushup that's ok. Muscles adapt rapidly, so every week or two add an extra pushup. There is no rule saying that pushups have to be consecutive either. Mix it up with 1 pushup every hour this weekend. The numbers can only increase as we continue for the rest of the year.

MOTIVATION & EARLY ALERTNESS PART 1:

Misery kills motivation. If we enjoy exercise, then we will do it consistently every day.

Light exercise can be very beneficial when we are overweight, if you find the right amount. There have been several times that I have walked up hills for 2 hours on warm days, only to return home completely exhausted.

Instead of something so exhausting, I now walk for 30 minutes on a cool morning. (It takes me about 25 minutes to walk a mile.) Afterwards, I feel prepared to conquer the day.

The reason I feel better after a morning walk is simple. First thing in the morning (or when we wake up), our blood is pumping slower. Do enough to pump that blood through your brain, and you should feel energized mentally.

But, this all depends on our bodies. Simply walk every day observing how tired you become. Every morning add or reduce the amount of exercise until you find the sweet spot.

After so many days or weeks, push yourself a little harder. Walk past a few more telephone poles, buildings, streets etc.

From time to time it might be good to push yourself to your limits. Though you may feel pain and exhaustion, there remains a great sense of pride when you take exercise to a new level.

If you are interested in how many miles you walk, there is a feet and mile tool on Google Earth.

MOTIVATION & EARLY ALERTNESS PART 2:

I am a big believer of waking up early. A sunrise feels energizing. By waking up at 5am-7am, we are ahead of the gates.

Why do we feel good early in the morning? It's a part of our circadian rhythm. In nature we would have to wake up for the morning sunlight.

Every night I prepare for tomorrows weather, so there's no surprises. I check the forecast in order to prepare my clothing accordingly.

If it's going to rain I place my mp3 player in a zip lock bag with a certain playlist set for my walk.

If you have machines that you never use, then I would recommend using one first thing in the morning to get the blood pumping through your brain on rainy days.

Whether its summer or winter, 5am is a great time to stay cool. Walking while it is snowing can add some fun to your walk too. Personally, I prefer fog walking.

TOO SHY TO WALK:

If you are concerned about people seeing you during a walk, I will show you the best times to avoid being noticed by people in your neighborhood. The following 3 graphs will identify the best hours to get outside without being recognized by the masses.

The information ahead is also useful to people with depression, & anxiety, as well as other mental illnesses that make it difficult to interact with the community. Times may vary on the weekends.

The best times to walk without too many people roaming around are [9am-2pm & 1am-6am]. I will explain why.

If you look at the chart labeled "Time Neighbors Wake Up" on the next page I created by merging two charts found online, you'll see that the first bar on the left represents midnight to 4am. Only 3% of the neighborhood is awake to see you during this time-frame.

The next bar is 4am-6am. On this time-frame 18% of the people are awake.

I imagine that most of these night owls/early-birds are too busy to notice you. Early birds are preparing for work or school. The night owls are most likely glued to a monitor or TV screen. One exception would have to be holidays. A walk on Labor Day might be crowded. However, for the entire winter, most people want to stay indoors with the windows closed. Colder months are great for sweating less as well.

In the summer, I go for cool walks around 6am. Occasionally I pass 2 nurses. I am less than a block away from a nursing home in case you are wondering. Also, depending on your area, you may have to pass kids at a bus stop. That all depends on what time your local schools start.

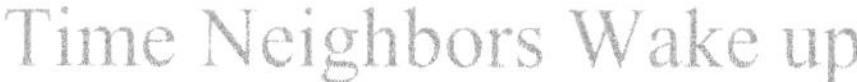

(3)(7)(6)

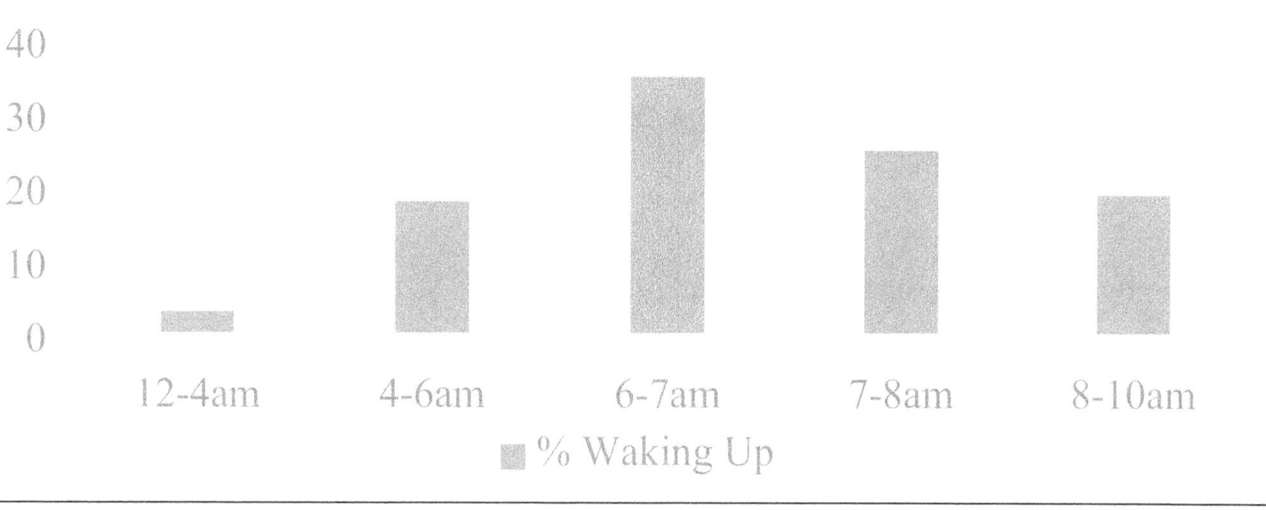

(4)(5)

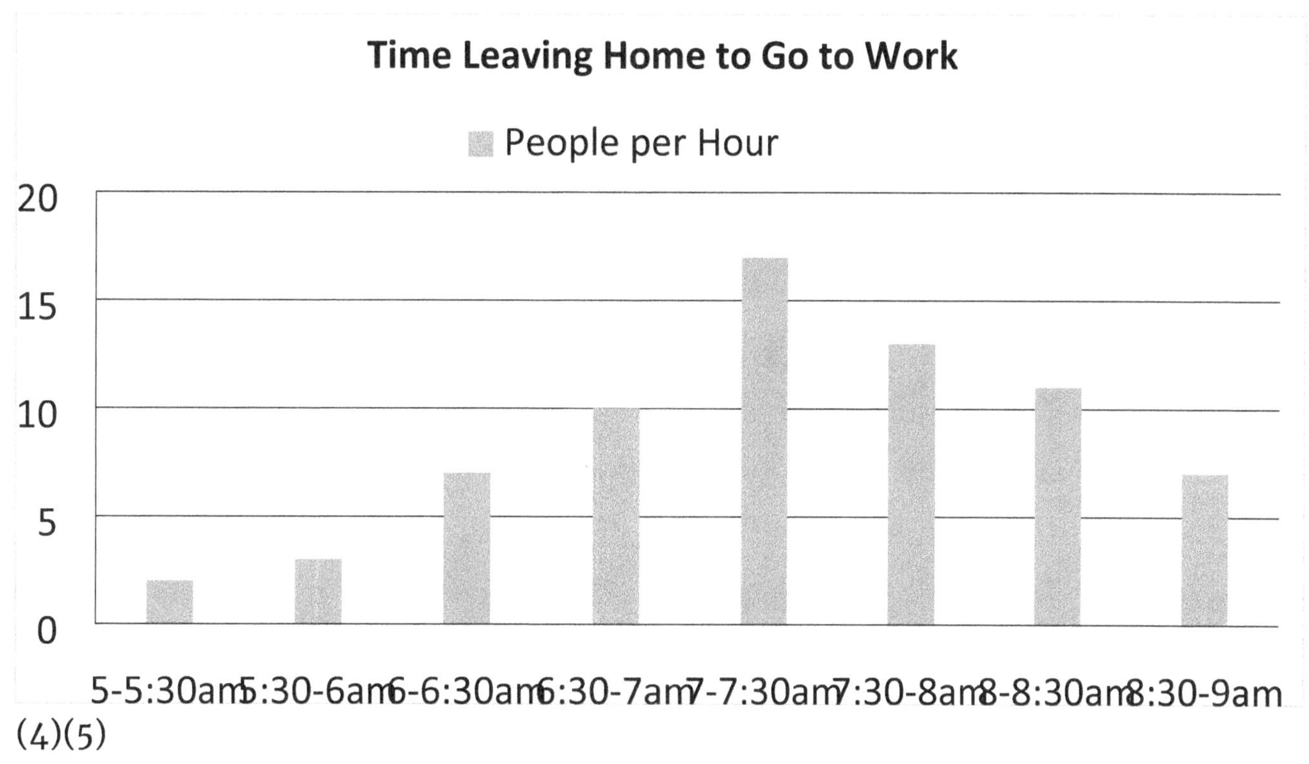

The next chart labeled "Time Leaving Home to Go to Work" is another amalgamation of statistics found on two separate websites. The number of people per hour totals 70 people.

Let's assume that everyone works for 8 hours a day. All 70 people have left from work by _**9am**_. A 5am person will leave work, and then go home 8 hours later at _**2pm**_. Therefore, our best window is _**9am-2pm**_.

The sweet spot is the midpoint at 11:30am. Between 11am-12pm my neighborhood is a ghost town when I walk my dog. During this time-frame there are hardly any dogs out to bark us too.

The two websites, for the 2nd graph, must not have found hours past 9am significant enough to mention.

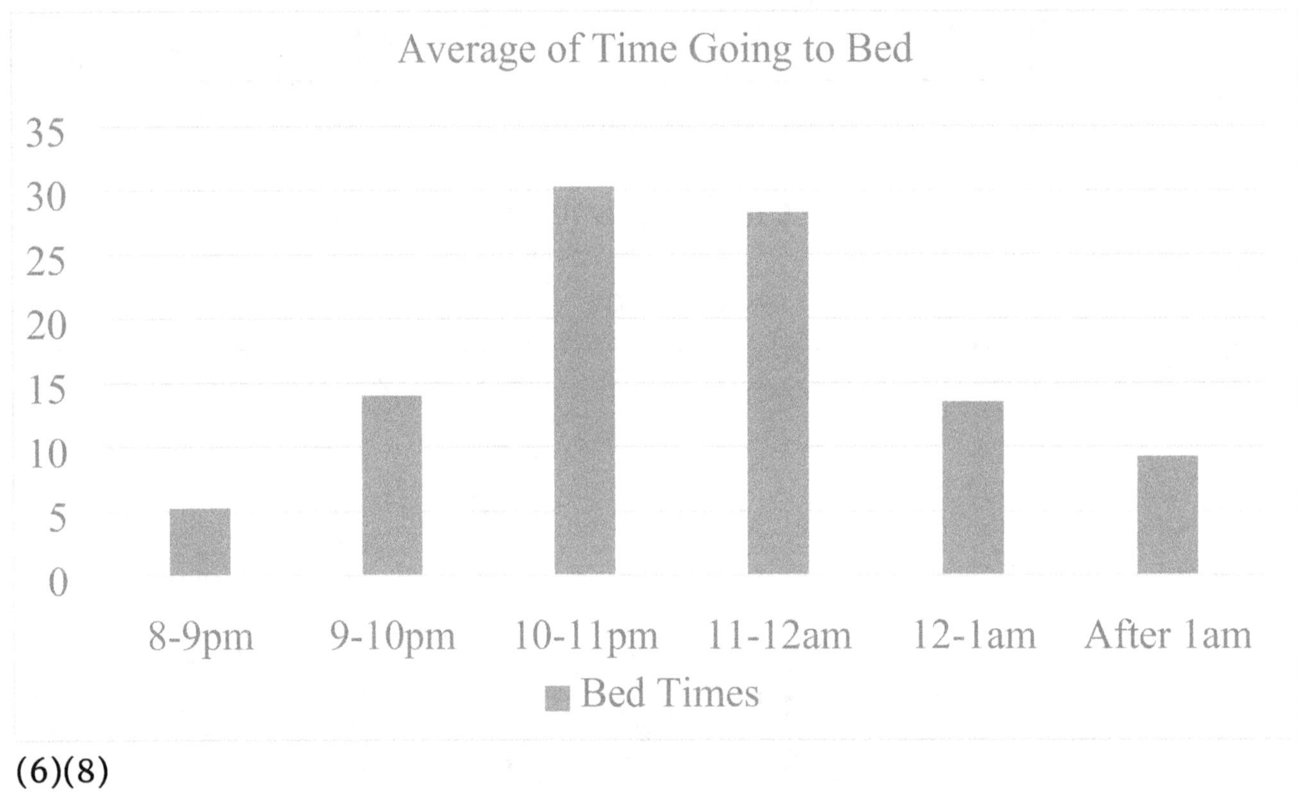

(6)(8)

We went over midnight to the afternoon. Let's be thorough by covering 8pm-after 1am, using two more charts in one.

According to the graph labeled "Average of Time Going to Bed", 78% of people are in bed by midnight. As long as you are not afraid of the dark, any time after 1am only leaves you vulnerable to the prying eyes of 9% of the neighborhood. Surely, most of those 9 percenter's awake at 1am are using computers, and not watching the streets.

HOME GYMS:

Al Roker, from The Today Show, shared his morning routine, partially consisting of a 30 minute walk on his home treadmill. Jessica Alba prefers to spin on a stationary bike.

Having gym equipment in the house is a great way to avoid bad weather. However, there are many house hold workout machines that will not help the shape, strength, or muscle growth we want to achieve. I highly recommend avoiding infomercial exercise machines.

There are 2 things to consider while selecting workout machines. Increasing heart rate (relative to breathing heavier) is one route to take. The other is to feel a strong sensation in your muscles. Two great examples of machines that elevate the heart rate includes, but is not limited to the treadmill & stationary bike.

Unless you are elderly, or going through rehabilitation, we need exercise equipment that makes us breathe more or have a burn in our muscles. Our muscles have to feel well used. There has to be a strong sensation similar to pain.

After some curls your muscles might feel stiff, lightweight, swollen, or sore. Muscles constantly change. The weak fibers die off, while the healthy muscle fibers continue to grow, or just plain survive. Bodybuilders understand this. They use specific workouts (just like the previous page) to keep the muscle fibers growing. Plenty of rest after workouts will also allow the muscle fibers to grow back.

If you are not used to soreness, it's not forever. Let's pretend that you get sore the day after doing some curls. Do those curls every day until the soreness in the muscle subsides. The discomfort lasts for about a week, then completely disappears. Now we can do that same workout every day without any more pain.

Our muscles adapt in a strange way that allows us to no longer experience any more soreness. But, if we stop doing the curl exercise for a month or two, then we must relive the pain when we start curling again.

The old saying goes, "no pain no gain".

When I was 10, my family couldn't afford much. So, when we were really strapped for cash, the next best thing would be a sack filled with dirt. Books come cheap in many sizes. I even used a small TV for lifts & an old mattress as a punching bag.

These days I use jump ropes and free weights. Jump ropes are very cheap while weights vary between $.50 & $1.00 per pound.

If you disagree with buying gym equipment, then using body weight as resistance will work just as well. This can be anything from balancing exercises to push-ups & sit-ups, to walking, jogging, boxing, pull-ups, crunches, etc. There are literally hundreds of exercises that do not require gym equipment. There are many apps out there as well, and we will go over some of them later.

Like I said, being overweight makes exercise much more difficult. If you don't like working out, then we can do one small exercise, like 5 sit-ups. Do 5 every day for a year and that is 1,825 sit-ups a year.

What if we skip the working out part? Can we simply stretch out? Yes! Besides the fact that we should learn to stretch before exercising anyways (prevents injuries & increases blood flow), stretching does not require so much of our heart rates. This is a great opportunity to build confidence with something every one of us is capable of.

In this book I cannot demonstrate stretching accurately. You'll have to Google some stretching videos. There are dozens of stretches to learn how to do.

Also, if you have a sedentary lifestyle, sitting up burns a lot more calories. Standing burns even more.

Additionally, if you weigh yourself right before & after sleep, you'll notice a 1-3 pound loss from sweat, body heat, and dead skin cells alone.

HEART RATES PART 1:

Following a high intensity workout means that you will need to know your MHR (Maximum Heart rate). Our individual MHR's are the highest amount of heart beats per minute (bpm) that we can safely handle during our cardio exercises.

Simply subtract your age from 220. I am 33 years old, so my initial bpm is 187. I should never reach 187bpm during cardio though. We only want 55-85% of our bpm number for 20-30 minutes of cardio. Therefore, my safe bpm for 20-30 minutes of cardio is 103-159bpm.

It's not hard to read your pulse. Use a 60 second watch/cell phone timer while counting your heart beats, by placing your index/middle finger on your wrist, or the side of your neck. Count the beats for 1 minute. Hence "beats per minute".

My heart can easily reach 200bpm if I push way too hard. I never attempt to reach 200bpm any longer. We can die from pushing ourselves like that.

A normal **resting** heart rate is 60-100bpm. Athletes can bring their **resting** heart rates well below 60bpm.

To measure a resting heart rate we check our pulse first thing in the morning. My resting heart rate is usually between 80-90bpm in the morning.

HEART RATES PART 2:

You should be wondering if the resting heart rate will go down if we lose weight. The answer is yes. Keeping track of our vitals should show a noticeable drop in bpm after a loss of about 30-50 pounds.

Many people in the online forums are reporting a drop of 20-40bpm after losing a significant amount of weight. However, it is unclear how much specific weight has to be dropped in order to lower a specific resting bpm.

I never recorded my own data for weight loss, but I witnessed my resting heart rate go down 40bpm after 6 months of quitting nicotine.

This information tells us that if we want to have an easier workout, we can diet to lower our resting bpm. Doing so will help us breathe better, and our hearts will not beat out of our chests so easily when we exercise.

Even so, I commend you for pushing past your limits if at all possible. Find what's right for you at the moment.

When I want high intensity exercise, I work a summer job landscaping, or picking up trash. If work is too hard, then I recommend going for a walk every morning, eating healthier, studying, and doing some exercises. Don't go a day without doing some of these things.

As they say, "do today what you will regret not doing tomorrow." Take baby steps if you have to.

SPRINTS:

"I can honestly attribute my abdominal development to my years as a high school & college sprint athlete", (13) says Obi Obadike (aka The Ripped Dude), host of more than 100 articles for fitness magazines and fitness websites.

People group abs differently. The basic way to look at our abs is by dividing them into upper and lower. Targeting the lower abs can be accomplished by crunching with our lower body. Sprinting is a perfect way of doing so, because of how high and fast the legs move. In a similar approach we target upper abs by crunching with our upper body. Ex, sit-ups & Crunches.

Again, in order for us to make exercise a routine we must work out enough to feel good, but not so much that we will give up altogether. After you establish a good routine, workout as hard as you like.

If you are pushing yourself too hard, then please remember to take some time off. Getting rest is sometimes more important for your body than the exercise alone.

BAD KNEES:

Bad knees deserve extra care. Perform leg raises, resistance band side steps, go for light walks, & try other leg lifts. All Squats are hard on the knees period. Do not perform lunges on bad knees either.

My Mom has had bad knees for several years now. She loves stationary bikes. Stationary bikes often times have resistance settings. You want low resistance with high reps. Do enough to raise your bpm.

Mom wants to do water aerobics someday too. Swimming pools are easy on most physical ailments as well. You're near weightless in the water, so you can move without the weight on your knees.

Some athletes even perform running drills in swimming pools. The elderly mainly want to get the blood flowing to their legs, otherwise the legs will swell. This is especially true for those elderly with a sedentary lifestyle and/or diabetes.

Where I live we have outdoor pools, an indoor pool, a wave pool, even a river. Some people even have lakes & beaches nearby. It's a great way to get out and get moving.

Yoga is great for strength rehabilitation of many body parts (including knees), and I have only heard good things from female acquaintances. I highly recommend giving yoga an effort. It's low intensity with long duration. Just don't push through too much pain. You can still get hurt.

DIET & NUTRITION:

CALORIES & CARBOHYDRATES:

Countless people restrict calories or carbs to lose weight. My high school classmates use to argue about which one to cut down on. The simple answer is that you can drop weight by reducing either one. However, we get more food options from using a moderation of both.

For instance, let's take a look at a well-balanced meal. We have half of a plate of spaghetti (high carb/low calorie) with a fillet of fish (low cal/low carb). Maybe some green beans too (low cal/low carb). A glass of milk will add extra calories, carbs, and nutrition. It's amazing how satiary (filling) this meal plan is.

That is a great variety with almost every section of the food pyramid. A well balanced meal will have low carbs & low calories. The only thing we are missing is some mixed nuts, or seeds. High calorie/Low carb.

Most meats (except seafood) are low carb/high calorie, while white (starchy) foods like potatoes & pasta are high carb/low calorie.

The healthiest example is a fillet of fish. Fish is extremely low in calories & low in carbs. Most colorful veggies are exceptionally low calorie/low carb as well. There is a list of negative calorie, low carb, and low calorie foods ahead.

BMR (BASAL METABOLIC RATE):

If you would like to know the amount of calories that you need to lose weight then you will need to know your __BMR__, aka the **Basal Metabolic Rate**. BMR is the number of calories you'd burn if you stayed in bed all day. The formula is:

Women: BMR = 655 + (4.35 x **weight** in pounds) + (4.7 x **height** in inches) - (4.7 x age in years)

Men: BMR = 66 + (6.23 x **weight** in pounds) + (12.7 x **height** in inches) - (6.8 x age in years)

There are simple & faster BMR calculators online that will do all of the work for you. If you want to do the math on your own, be sure to use PEMDAS. Do everything in parenthesis 1st. Next do addition & finally subtraction.

My BMR is 1957. Next we use the **Harris Benedict Equation** to factor in how much energy we burn through work and exercise using one of the following:

- If you are sedentary (little or no exercise) : Calorie-Calculation = BMR x 1.2

- If you are lightly active (light exercise/sports 1-3 days/week) : Calorie-Calculation = BMR x 1.375

- If you are moderately active (moderate exercise/sports 3-5 days/week) : Calorie-Calculation = BMR x 1.55

- If you are very active (hard exercise/sports 6-7 days a week) : Calorie-Calculation = BMR x 1.725

- If you are extra active (very hard exercise/sports & physical job or 2x training) : Calorie-Calculation = BMR x 1.9

I work on a computer & walk 2 miles a day at best, so I will multiply my BMR (1,957) by 1.375 = 2,690. 2,690 is the total number of calories I need in order to **maintain** my current weight.

Let's look at the extreme. "When you're on a low-calorie diet, you usually get between 800 and 1,500 calories a day", States Registered &Licensed Dietician, Christine

Mikstas, in an article for WebMD. The average weight loss will be 44 pounds over 12 weeks. (17)

Men will be closer to 1,500 calories a day to lose weight. It really depends on sex and height.

WHAT IS A CARBOHYDRATE?

(1g of carbohydrates equals 4 calories.)(4 calories do not have to contain 1g of carbs though.) The carbohydrate gets its name from the molecule $(CH_2O)n$. While a calorie is the measurement of energy, the carb is the matter in food itself.

Both can result into additional body fat, unless it is burnt through exercise and digestion.

Carbohydrates are turned into the same substance as table sugar once digested. Both sugars are broken down to be sent through the bloodstream for the body to use as energy. Excessive blood sugar will be stored in the liver and the body's fat cells.

COMPLEX CARBOHYDRATES:

Complex carbs are digested slowly, keeping you fueled longer. You will find more nutrition in complex carbohydrates as well. They include; whole grains, fruits, vegetables, nuts, etc.

SIMPLE CARBOHYDRATES:

Simple Carbohydrates are the ones that are most obvious to avoid. This includes: Cakes, cookies, pies, sugary cereals, soda's, etc. These are the ones that cause the blood sugar to spike the most.

On the Next Five Pages are lists of (Negative Calorie), (Low Carbohydrate), & (Low Calorie) Foods.

NEGATIVE CALORIE FOODS:

Negative calorie foods take more calories to burn, than they actually contain.

Apples
Leek
Lettuce
Onion
Orange
Peppers
Pineapple
Plum
Raspberries
Spinach
Strawberries
Tomatoes
Watermelon
Apricots
Asparagus
Beet
Broccoli
Cauliflower
Carrots
Celery
Cranberries
Cucumber
Grapefruit
Green bean

LOW CARBOHYDRATE FOODS:

Eggs
Fats
Fish
Fruits
High-fat dairy
Meat
Nuts and seeds
Vegetable

LOW CALORIE FOODS:

Apple
Apricot
Artichoke
Asparagus
Avocado
Bamboo Shoots
Banana
Bean Sprouts
Beans
Beets
Bell Peppers
Blackberries

Blueberries
Broccoli
Brussels sprouts
Cabbage
Cantaloupe
Carrots
Cauliflower
Celery
Cherries
Coconuts
Collard Greens
Corn
Cranberries
Cucumber
Dates
Eggplant
Figs
Garlic
Gooseberries
Grapefruit
Grapes
Green Beans
Greens
Honeydew Melon
Kale
Kiwifruit
Leeks
Lemons
Lettuce

Lima Beans
Limes
Mandarin Oranges
Mangos
Mushrooms
Nectarines
Okra
Onion
Oranges
Papayas
Peaches
Peas
Peppers
Pineapple
Plantains
Plums
Pomegranate
Potatoes
Pear
Prunes
Pumpkin
Radishes
Raisins
Raspberries
Red Cabbage
Lettuce
Spinach
Sprouts
Strawberries

String Beans
Sweet Potato (Yam)
Tangerines
Tomato
Turnip
Water Chestnuts
Watercress
Watermelon
Squash

AVOIDING SUGAR:

Staying away from sugar will make weight loss magnitudes easier. The weight will fall off gradually, just from giving up sweets.

It takes patience to quit sugar. Every time you fail, take a break. Stop trying hard for a while. Just do not quit altogether.

The best substitutions for sugar are more natural sugars like fruit. Fruit is a much healthier sugar. Blood sugar will not crash as much. Also, there are more nutrients, as well as fiber. I could eat 6 oranges a day and still lose weight.

The biggest problem I had with sugar was that it is extremely cheap. I've seen 1 pound of sugar sell for 50 cents before. And it's easy. Snack cakes, cookies and pies are ready to eat from the box.

Again, medications can cause an increase in sugar cravings as well, so beware. Sugar will cause more hunger too.

Now, if you would like to become a lean bodybuilder then you want to avoid sugar altogether. That includes carbs that can be converted into sugars; such as potatoes, rice, flour, corn, or other grains & fruits.

However, most of us are not bodybuilding enthusiasts. We want to take the necessary steps to lose weight while feeling better with a happier, healthier lifestyle. Yeah?

Quitting sugar can be difficult, but withdrawal symptoms are very minor compared to other addictions. What really helps is a couple of supplement pills at the end of this book. All of the supplements have changed my life.

I feel that the extra supplement Chasteberry is worth mentioning, because all of them help me on a daily basis. I've experimented with about 100 supplements for weeks and months at a time, and only a few of them were proven to work well for me. That's for later, so let's move on.

FATS; GOOD VS BAD:

It's helpful to know one Latin word to sort the Good fats from the bad fats. The Latin root word "un" means "not". (Ex. Un-happy= not happy) One of our bad fats on the label is called saturated fat. One good fat is **poly-<u>un</u>-saturated** fat. The other good fat is **mono-<u>un</u>-saturated** fat. In other words, our healthy fats have the root word "un", standing for "not" saturated.

Unsaturated fats are good for your heart & arteries, while saturated/Tran's fats cause clogged arteries & heart disease. Another real risk with fat is that foods with higher bad fat content tend to have more calories, causing weight gain.

The best examples of healthy fats are avocados, cheese, dark chocolate, eggs, fish, & nuts.

There is one fat we rarely see called Tran's fat. Tran's fats are mainly found in fried foods, and red meats, including whey protein powders. I prefer to stay away from these, because they are the worst fats, but I never turn down a free burger.

CHOLESTEROL; GOOD VS BAD:

Cholesterol is very simple to sort out. Good cholesterol is found in any seafood and white meats. Eggs are another great choice. Doctors use to tell us that the yolk of the egg was high in cholesterol. That statement is true. However, we now know that egg yolks have the good cholesterol. Good cholesterol will even help us lower our bad cholesterol. The cholesterol you want to avoid is mostly found in red meats, fried foods, and most protein powders have bad cholesterol as well.

Bad cholesterol (LDL) causes heart disease by clogging your arteries. The exact opposite is true for good cholesterol. Good cholesterol (HDL) sweeps bad cholesterol away.

HDL & LDL will not be on the nutrition fact label. At least, as I am writing this in Nov, 2018 you will only see the word "cholesterol" on food labels. Just remember that seafood, eggs, and white meats are the healthy meats. No batter or breading either.

Doctors test HDL & LDL levels. Just in case you need to know the difference between HDL & LDL, remember H for heaven. ***(HDL)*** is the place you want to go. L is the Lower place you don't want to visit. ***(LDL)***

SALT & SWEETENERS:

Artificial sweeteners can aid in cutting calories as long as they are used in moderation.

Artificial sweeteners may cause excess hunger, but they cannot be broken down enough to be digested. This means that people will not gain weight as a direct result of the artificial sweetener.

Be wary of sugar free foods though. The real risk with artificial sweetener is that people think that they can eat as much as they want. That is false. Many sugar free items contain high amounts of carbs with little to no nutrition.

When we look at the nutritional facts on the label of diet soda cans, we notice that there is nothing but large amounts of sodium. Therefore, you are drinking mostly salt water. Black salt water if you enjoy the dark kind. Keep in mind that excessive sodium can cause water weight.

Sedentary diabetics will have swollen legs with open sores from too much fluid. Gravity brings the fluid down to the legs. If this person does not walk much, then the fluid never gets pumped back up, so the legs continue to swell. Salt makes this condition worse.

If this happens to someone you know, the legs need exercised and be kept up while resting. Avoid salty processed foods and soda as well.

GLYCEMIC INDEX:

The GI rating found on the nutritional facts labels consist of a scale of 1-100. The lower G.I number for a food (55 or less) means that after consumption, the carbs will digest slowly; creating a slow, steady increase in blood sugar. The lower the G.I number, the better it is for you.

Higher G.I numbers (56-100) will cause a sudden blood sugar spike, making you feel full, but then you'll feel hungry again after the blood sugar takes a sudden crash. The G.I numbers on food labels are valuable for diabetics. Slower, steadier blood sugar levels can be a great way to feel full longer for anyone though.

ATKINS DIET:

Atkins is low in carbs with high fatty proteins.

Foods to Eat on Atkins: Meats, Seafood, Eggs, kale, spinach, broccoli, asparagus, butter, cheese, cream, fat yogurt, nuts and seeds, extra virgin olive oil, coconut oil, water, coffee, tea & avocados.

Foods to Avoid on Atkins: Sugar, grains, & Tran's fats.

Avoid the following at first: high carb vegetables, fruits, potatoes, sweet potatoes, lentils, beans, chickpeas etc.

MEAT DIET:

As I stated before, we can encounter so many more food options if we eat a combination of low Cal/mid carb foods, with low carb/mid Cal foods. However, eating mostly meat will still result in weight loss.

This greasy method is not healthy at all. It's a diet that allows you to eat foods with artery clogging cholesterol yeah?

I'm not going to judge anyone. Honestly, this is worth trying out. I have lost weight many times this way when my budget was small. Hotdogs are cheap after all. Who knows, this might be what you need temporarily.

KETOSIS:

Ketosis is a means of burning body fat by eating very few carbs. 50 grams or less per day. When we do not consume enough carbs, our body's resort to burning stored up fat. It can be dangerous if you're sick, diabetic, or pregnant though.

WebMD's Michael Dansinger, MD says that "For healthy people who don't have diabetes and aren't pregnant, ketosis usually kicks in after 3 or 4 days of eating less than 50 grams of carbohydrates per day." (1)

Is Ketosis Safe:

There are many studies finding that ketosis is safe for severely overweight individuals, but the weight tends to come back within a year.

It's easy to realize why the weight comes back. I have been on both low calorie & low carb diets. (Ketosis being low carb.) There is a rebound effect. We have to quit ketosis at some point. I mean we can't lose weight forever. So what's the game plan for when we stop the low carb diet? We only have one choice after any diet comes to an end. We have to eat healthy. If we don't learn to eat healthy, we only have our old habits.

Best foods for Ketosis:

The best foods for ketosis are: any meat/seafood, vegetables, eggs, oils, cheese, etc.

SOME OF MY FAVORITE FOODS:

I suggest exploring different foods for the rest of your life. If you like 5 new healthy foods every year, 10 years later you will have 50 healthy foods to add to your new lifestyle.

As a snack, I am really into Jif Fat Reduced peanut butter from Walmart. Surprisingly, fat reduced doesn't stick in my mouth as much. For some reason it tastes better by itself too.

Another snack I buy is corn chips. I choose them, because they are not the tastiest chips available. This prevents me from over eating them. The corn chips also give me the fat I crave every now and then.

If you are going to eat junk food, then tone down the intensity of the flavor. Instead of cookies, buy animal crackers. Instead of Dorito's, buy chees-its.

Sometimes I buy 60 eggs, so that I can bake them in the oven. There are several egg recipes out there. My favorite one is to put 2 cans of mixed vegetables in a casserole dish (drain water out first). I sprinkle shredded cheese on top. I add at least 12 beat eggs, and cover the eggs with more cheese. The dish bakes for 25 minutes. It takes 15 minutes to prepare, and less than 45 minutes total, for enough meals that lasts' 3-4 days.

Ranch dressing is excellent for dipping vegetables. I enjoy dipping raw baby carrots in ranch. Even the stems of broccoli taste good in ranch (FYI, baby carrots are not grown. They are cut from the large carrots.)

Healthy cereals are the "green eggs & ham" of the real world. Most of my life I rejected the thought of eating healthy cereal. However, I kept forcing down bran flakes, Cheerios, and plain Rice Crispies. Now I love them all.

Other favorites of mine include; nuts, fruits, fried fish, flavored crackers…

I enjoy junk food about twice a month. My favorite is a half a gallon of chocolate milk. It will not last a day in my fridge. I even go to an all you can eat buffet once every couple of months. If I'm going to eat big, then that will be my only meal for the day.

Below are just a few snacks low on calories, carbs, or sugar to begin with. Keep reading labels to create a list you can call your own.

S F Pudding (60Cal/13Carb)

Pork Rinds (154Cal/0Carb)

Olives (115Cal/6Carb)

Pickles (4Cal/1Carb)

Almonds (163Cal/12Carb)

Pretzels (109Cal/23Carb)

Cheese-Its (150Cal/17Carb)

Peanut Butter (190Cal/8Carb)

Raisins (129Cal/34Carb)

Banana Chips (147Cal/17Carb)

Pickled Eggs (79Cal/1Carb)

Cheese Cubes x1 (16Cal/.1Carb)

Pepperoncini's (15 Cal/4Carb)

Jerky (82Cal/2Carb)

SMOOTHIES:

Many TV series have shown characters with a look of disgust on their faces as they drink a green smoothie. It's not like that at all. Smoothies are often sweet & fruity (even if you add a vegetable to the mix).

There's a smoothie I prepare all year. It consists of frozen juice, frozen chunks of bananas, Soy Protein mix, peanut butter, and cold water from the fridge, blended with a teaspoon of 0 Cal sweetener.

The blender I use is a $25 Farberware one from Walmart that blends everything inside each plastic drinking glass. It should come with 4 tall plastic drinking cups, blade attachments & two smaller cups. The blades rinse clean, plus there's no giant pitcher to clean up after like the old traditional blenders. Fill the cups with water to soak or wash the cups right away, and they will not be difficult to clean.

If the shake doesn't want to mix, then try placing the ingredients in a different order. Often times my fruit sticks to the bottom, so I stir everything before screwing the blade attachment on.

There is no need for ice if you keep all of the ingredients in the freezer. I break bananas into quarters & place them in the freezer. They will last about 3-5 months. 25

bananas last me about a month. Bananas are ridiculously cheap if you buy them right before they go bad.

I also freeze juice in ice cube trays. Making the juice from frozen concentrate is probably the cheapest way with no added sugars.

I drink shakes every day and I pay under $35 for the entire month for the frozen juice cubes, bananas, sweetener, soy protein, and peanut butter.

If you dare, add some spinach or nuts to the mix. The blender is also great for iced drinks.

I tried kale in a smoothie once. I'm a big believer in trying new foods until they taste good, except for kale. I doubt if I will ever enjoy kale. I suppose we all have one food we will never enjoy.

WATER:

Water is the greatest change you can make to your diet. It takes a lot of practice, especially because water taste terrible first thing in the morning, and when it is warm. What helps is to keep two jugs of cold water in the fridge. That way, when one is empty, you will still have a cold jug. Possibly swish some mouthwash in the morning before drinking water too.

Force yourself to drink water. Try to drink a dozen glasses of water per week and you will get used to it. I always hated water, but now I live on it. Sometimes I drink nothing but water every day for an entire week or two.

Trust me. Force 1 glass of water down every day for an entire month. In my opinion there's no need for putting lemon in it either. Although, other people claim lemon water is the way to go.

The correct quantity of water a day can be remembered by the 8x8 rule. This means 8-eight ounce glasses of water, or ½ a gallon. Each glass is smaller than a can of soda.

If you can do this every day, great. On a slow day I drink at least a gallon of water. Drinking water can curb your appetite as well.

As a warning, water at fast food outlets is terrible. At McDonalds they gave me a large ice water, but charged me for a large tea. The water came right from the faucet?! Meanwhile, the person I went with was charged less than my water for a bucket of coke. Their OJ is tiny. Their milk isn't any better. It is a shame that we have to over pay for something that was free in the 1990's.

PORTION CONTROL:

Honestly, the correct portions of food can be disappointing. In most cases, serving sizes on food labels will be less than what we normally eat. For me, I use to have a **big** glass of milk with my **full** bowl of cereal. Once I began paying attention to serving sizes, I discovered that I had to start eating a measuring cup of cereal with only a measuring cup of milk.

When I first started dieting, I concentrated on eating smaller portions. It takes practice. Over the years I learned that portion control is just a minor component of what we need to keep the weight off. When portion control fails, try a day of ketosis. After ketosis, focus on lowering calories. When low cal foods get tough, drink a smoothie or two every day. Or, mix and match the other weight loss methods.

Smaller portions can be made much simpler if you have well balanced meals. Every item adds up on the plate.

If you are not ready & willing to try balanced meals, then I recommend starting out by keeping the correct portions of just one of your favorite foods daily. Work your way up.

You'll need to use the correct serving size for each item to understand the numbers on the nutritional facts label. If you are doubling the serving size, then you have to double the calories, fats, sodium etc.

FAST FOODS:

The objective of every fast food place is to keep you coming back. This is accomplished by adding as much fat, or sugar to your meals as possible. In a report in gizmodo.com,

Annalee Newitz explains how "some fast foods have the hormone ghrelin mixed in food, causing your brain to react to food in the same way that addicts respond to drugs". (14)

Avoiding fast food is imperative to losing weight. The fast food habit only takes 3 weeks to officially overcome. Eating TV dinners in place of fast food makes it really easy to break the fast food habits.

I still eat out when someone invites me. Maybe even to celebrate a big event, but I don't go out every day like I use to.

If you are going to eat fast food, I recommend bean burritos at Taco Bell, something from the healthy spectrum at Subway, or McDonald's sausage burritos. The sausage burrito has eggs, sausage bits, cheese, & bell pepper. Believe me when I tell you that the sausage burrito is one of their lowest calorie items at 300 calories each (In 2018).

DIABETES:

A person of any age can become a type 2 diabetic. The chances of getting type 2 diabetes increases as you exercise less & gain weight. Losing weight can reverse type 2 diabetes, especially through eating right combined with exercise.

The following is how type 2 diabetes occurs. Sugar causes a blood sugar spike. Insulin is produced in the pancreas to handle the blood sugar. Eventually, we eat so much over the years that our liver fills with extra blood sugar. The pancreas cannot produce enough insulin and stops working. Once the body can't produce enough insulin, we have to treat our diabetes with insulin shots 3 times a day.

The finger prick will test your blood sugar levels. That information lets the Doctor know how many units of insulin you need in each syringe. Finger pricks will also let you know when to take insulin shots or when you need to eat due to low blood sugar.

I guarantee that if you walk 10-30 minutes a day, stay away from the sweets 28 days out of the month, and learn to eat healthier, you will steadily lose weight. (Giving up sweets alone will facilitate weight loss greatly). After accomplishing these methods over the years, not only will your doctor be happy, but most likely you may not have type 2 diabetes anymore.

If you are obese and do not think that you are diabetic, just remember that we can have diabetes for years without even knowing it. My Aunt (God rest her soul) was overweight for almost a decade before collapsing to the floor inside of a Kroger's, due to hypoglycemia. After that incident, she had to take insulin 3 times a day for the rest of her life.

Unfortunately, people with diabetes need to have the right amount of carbohydrates per meal. That being 45-60 grams. (Diabetics need 130-230 grams of carbs per day altogether.) Inadequate carbs will cause the unpleasant hypoglycemia symptoms, including but not limited to; sweating, feeling faint, going into a coma, and even death. Hyperglycemia happens when a diabetic has too much blood sugar, hypoglycemia stems from blood sugar that is too low. Both are serious.

For people with diabetes, look for the healthier, complex carbohydrate options such as fruits, veggies, and whole grains. Another great option is fish. Just remember that fish has no carbs, so we need to add foods with 45-60g of carbs. Ex. fruit, colorful vegetables, or a potato.

FALL HUNGER:

The concept of fall season hunger is not well known. This is my 5th year noticing this problem. Not everyone is going to have it. But, like me, you may have had this problem your whole life, without ever realizing the extra hunger cravings (pangs) every year right around the fall season.

It's reasonable that every living thing in my area has to prepare body fat for the cold season. My fall hunger occurs from mid-September to mid-November. Nothing (not even pills) will stop the cravings entirely.

Right now there are not many resources about fall hunger on the internet. The best that can be done is damage control. If you're losing 3 pounds a month, then from September 15th to November 15th we almost certainly have to settle for maintaining the weight we have. This year I settled for an increase of 8 pounds, plus the two months afterwards, it had taken to lose it again.

Just recognizing fall hunger can be beneficial. It allows us to see what we are about to run into in time to hit the brakes. If you don't have this in mind then it's easy to coast into over-eating, gaining weight, & losing confidence again.

USEFUL INFORMATION:

REBOUND EFFECT (AKA RELAPSE):

Most people relapse into gaining the weight back shortly after their first success. Relapse comes at any time. When it occurs, we can't get on with our lives without that tempting food luring us back in. It's as if we are flies near a bug zapper.

After the 2 years it had taken me to officially quit smoking, something was wrong. I couldn't free myself of the nagging questions in my mind. "What happens if I smoke again?", "Would it be the same?", "Could it be like my first time?", "Maybe I can control it better?" The same is true for dieting. What if I have 1 more cookie? 1 soda? 1 candy bar?

Not every habit is so terrible. You might not ask these questions in the back of your mind. Something in your life might be the trigger. Perhaps you can't sleep at night and a late night snack is tempting. It could be a lost job, or you get sad & lonely. Similar feelings are worthy enough for us to try to justify feeling better with food. Reaching our weight loss goal can even be the trigger.

Once I went 2 years without any caffeine, my sister was moving in with me. I had no clue if we would get along. I was so used to living alone, that my sister moving in was extra stressful for me. She left her pop in the fridge. After she was gone, I stared at her cold pop. It drew me in closer. By the end of the day I had to buy her another 6-pack. Sadly, I drank that too.

When relapse happens, we quickly learn that we need to do more than lose weight. We must be able to keep it off. In order to do that, we must learn to eat healthy throughout our daily lives.

Not learning to eat healthy will lead to a relapse. And often times relapse is part of the process. It happens to the best of us.

I learned in a ropes course class that if we cross a bridge halfway, it is just as far to walk forward as it is to give up and turn back. Relapse can sometimes be considered a halfway point across our bridge.

THE FIRST FEW MONTHS:

Have you ever lost a successful amount of weight in the beginning, only to plateau, or barely lose anything in the following months?

Your first two months will likely be your most successful months. The reason is that overeating cause's body tissue to retain water. Therefore, eating healthier (less salt) sheds what some call "water weight" during the first 2-3 months' of dieting.

Also, for the first month of exercise, most people will gain weight, even though they are eating healthy. This happens to Hollywood actors often. Be patient. Your muscles are dying and fat is burning. The body goes into panic mode for the first few weeks and needs extra sustenance to heal. After a few weeks you'll start to shed weight again.

WHEN TO WEIGH IN:

We are all different when it comes to how often we should weigh ourselves. Weighing daily is not for everyone.

Most people cannot handle watching the numbers increase. Be realistic. The numbers on the scale will not go down every day. Often times I have gained weight on the days I felt skinny, and lost weight on days I felt fat. It took me years of success & failure to feel perfectly comfortable checking my weight on a day to day basis.

Using the scale after eating sweets is tricky. I never gain weight right away after treating myself to chocolate milk. The weight tags on 2-3 days later! The scale can mess with most people's heads, especially when you are more anxious to lose weight.

Whether we weigh ourselves once a day; every two weeks, or once a month, we need a weighing routine. We should wear roughly the same weight in clothing when we weigh ourselves. Sometimes I will take advantage of using the toilet first as well. That might sound like cheating, but it's a routine that allows me to be consistent every month. Choosing the best weight of the last 3 days at the calendar month can add some whimsy to your weigh-in too. Just be as consistent as possible. You don't have to use the toilet btw.

PATIENCE:

Again, patience is the key to success. Try creating a 1 year plan to lose 3 pounds every month. That adds up to 36 pounds a year. When we turn our small goals into a 5 year plan something incredible happens. The product of 5x36 makes 180 Pounds in 5 years!

Think of the little changes possible to achieve your 5 year plan. (Maybe set additional goals to your 5 year plan as well.) You could even go as far as to spend 2 years learning how to lose weight and spend that time experimenting with what you've learned. After 2 years, get serious with all of your discoveries.

WEIGHT CHARTS (MEN & WOMEN):

I have created two sets of weight charts from different sources on the following pages. The sources are the weight charts for men & women in the Armed Forces plus the weight chart from the National Institutes of Health.

Ex. Let's say you are a 4' 10" tall male. You should weigh somewhere in between 91-118 as an ideal athletic weight. For the Army (Where you need strong muscle mass) you should weight around 91-132.

These numbers are very useful. I am 5'9". 168 is the most I should weigh to be fit. 186 is what I should weight to have the strength & endurance that the US Army requires. Whereas, if I have bad knees it is probably best to have as little weight on my haunches as possible. That's when 128 pounds could be handy.

<u>**Below is the Men's Weight Chart based on Height. (10) (11)**</u>

<u>**(Height)(Min Weight)(Ideal Max Weight-Max Army)**</u>

<u>**(4' 10") (91) (118-132)**</u>

<u>**(4' 11") (94) (123-137)**</u>

<u>**(5') (97) (127-141)**</u>

<u>**(5' 1") (100) (131-146)**</u>

<u>**(5' 2") (104) (135-150)**</u>

<u>**(5' 3") (107) (140-155)**</u>

<u>**(5' 4") (110) (144-160)**</u>

<u>**(5' 5") (114) (149-165)**</u>

<u>**(5' 6") (117) (154-170)**</u>

<u>**(5' 7") (121) (158-176)**</u>

<u>**(5' 8") (125) (163-181)**</u>

<u>**(5' 9") (128) (168-186)**</u>

<u>**(5' 10") (132) (173-192)**</u>

<u>**(5' 11") (136) (178-197)**</u>

<u>**(6') (140) (183-203)**</u>

<u>**(6' 1") (144) (188-208)**</u>

<u>**(6' 2") (148) (193-214)**</u>

<u>**(6' 3") (152) (199-220)**</u>

<u>**(6' 4") (156) (204-226)**</u>

<u>**(6' 5") (160) (218-232)**</u>

<u>**(6' 6") (164) (223-238)**</u>

(6' 7") (168) (229-244)

(6' 8") (173) (234-250)

Below is the Women's Weight Chart based on Height. (10) (12)

(Height) (Min Weight) (Ideal Max Weight-Max Army)

(4' 10") (91) (118-124)

(4' 11") (94) (123-128)

(5') (97) (127-133)

(5' 1") (100) (131-137)

(5' 2") (104) (135-142)

(5' 3") (107) (140-146)

(5' 4") (110) (144-151)

(5' 5") (114) (149-156)

(5' 6") (117) (154-161)

(5' 7") (121) (158-166)

(5' 8") (125) (163-171)

(5' 9") (128) (168-176)

(5' 10") (132) (173-181)

(5' 11") (136) (178-186)

(6') (140) (183-191)

(6' 1") (144) (188-197)

(6' 2") (148) (193-202)

(6' 3") (152) (199-208)

(6' 4") (156) (204-213)

(6' 5") (160) (210-219)

(6' 6") (164) (216-225)

(6' 7") (168) (221-230)

(6' 8") (173) (227-236)

GASTRIC BYPASS SURGERY:

Most people are familiar with this option. The stomach is reduced in size, making it possible for people to feel full faster. It's a serious surgery for those who are obese. Doctors will decide if the benefits outweigh the risks. Even with the surgery you must continue with better eating habits.

As of 2017, gastric bypass surgery costs $15,000 to $25,000 on average according to the National Institute of Diabetes & Digestive & Kidney Diseases. (15)

Insurance will cover part of any modern weight loss surgery. Anything considered experimental is not covered.

WEIGHT LOSS IMPLANT:

This is an implant placed in the abdomen, sending pulses to the brain through the vagus nerve to reduce hunger.

According to WebMD, a website with articles written by Doctors, "The FDA approved the device for the treatment of obese adults who have a body mass index (BMI) of at least 40, and for those with a BMI of at least 35 who have an obesity-related condition, such as high blood pressure or high cholesterol. Candidates are supposed to have tried to lose weight in a supervised weight-management program within the previous 5 years." (16)

To find your bmi, it is simplest to google "bmi calculator".

The 2017 implant cost was in the range of $20,000-$25,000. (16)

DRUGS THAT CAUSE WEIGHT GAIN:

Drugs can be the cause of sudden weight gain, and there are many. I've had a few different pills causing excessive hunger over the years. If you have more cravings, or sudden weight gain, make an appointment with your prescribing Doctor, and research your meds on WebMD by looking through a list of side effects and drug interactions.

If weight gain is a side effect of a prescription, then your Doctor can either give you a drug that can fight the side effect, or there may be another medication to replace it with.

It is also important to have your thyroid checked. An underactive thyroid has the same symptom of weight gain.

USEFUL FACTS:

Have you ever had trouble breathing while laid back after a meal? Over-eating can cause acid reflux. Most likely, this is what you are feeling. You become so full, that the food comes back up when you lie down.

Brushing your teeth during the last few hours of the day can help stop cravings. The idea is that we will not want to lose our fresh breathe by eating again.

If you have trouble sleeping, then it is a good idea not to eat during the last few hours before your bed time. I still have this problem at times. I think that I will go to sleep right after eating. Nope. The food makes me more alert from the digestion. Next thing I know I'm still awake two hours later.

SUPPLEMENTS:

(Please consult with your Doctor before trying these)
(Also check drug interactions & side effects at WebMD.com)

<u>Gymnema Syvestre</u>: This is a supplement that helps me stay away from sweets and fatty junk foods. I take 400mg twice daily. (This supplement might not work during fall hunger months).

While it is so much easier for me to stay away from junk food, there are times that I do treat myself. I might buy 1 candy bar a month. Possibly a half a gallon of chocolate milk once a month as well.

During the holidays my sister makes rum balls, so out of respect I like to eat as many as I like. Who wants to turn down a rum ball anyway? With birthdays I am the same way, but one piece of cake is my limit.

<u>Hoodia Gordonii</u>: While Gymnema Syvestre lowers sugar and fat cravings; Hoodia Gordonii helps me eat less often. Both supplements work best right before meals.

It has had one study with promising results. From www.globalhealingcenter.com **Dr. Edward** mentions in a 2015 article that Dr. Richard M. Goldfarb conducted a 28 day study in which, "participants experienced, on average, a 3.3% reduction in body weight, and a median weight loss of 10 pounds." (2)

<u>Chasteberry:</u> is just one more I want to throw in. It has nothing to do with weight loss, but if you are/or have a young man with too high of a libido, then I'm here to inform you that this will drop a man's libido by about 2/3. It was used as pepper in churches for thousands of years to help leaders keep their celibacy.

Note: I feel as though I cannot live without any of these 3 supplements. I have two Kroger bags of supplements I have experimented with over the years, but only these 3 have been life altering. This book is an educational tool. However, I would have a much more difficult time losing weight without the Hoodia Gordonii & Gymnema Syvestre.

Chasteberry has been a great success on my YouTube channel. There are thousands of people attracted to my Chasteberry video every year. Especially, since so many young men are addicted to pornography these days.

APPS:

Out of the many great apps available I have one for tracking weight loss called Simple Weight Tracker. It's one of the simpler apps I have. I enter my weight at the beginning of every month. The app places that number on a line graph for a better visual reference. Simply yeah?

I do not always cook big healthy meals, but when I feel like cooking something new I use the FitMenCook app. It allows me to create an organized grocery list after deciding on one of the 500 recipes. Just select the grocery icon, then unselect each item that you already have before you go to the store.

Another app I like is goal tracker. If you're quitting a bad habit, or trying something new, this app creates a calendar for every goal you want to keep track of. If you give up on eating ice cream, type in "quit ice cream", then every day mark that calendar with an X if you ate ice cream, or mark with a check if you didn't eat ice cream. It's that simple. If you forget to add a check, the app lets you add that check any time you feel like it.

There are many calorie counting apps available. The app will store the calories from your foods and it will save all of the meals you enter. I have counted carbs and calories by pen & paper. These apps make it so much simpler, and faster to keep track of your target calories.

Countless exercise/workout apps are out there, depending on what you want to try. Some of them show you how to perform the exercises. Others can customize your workouts. Some apps count your steps. You can find apps specific to your gender. There are 7 minute workouts, and 10 minute workouts. You can target specific areas such as; abs, upper body, or legs. Just search for what you want to try and learn about. Whatever doesn't work out might not be the best thing right now. Simply set aside what fails & search for the next app that may suit your needs better. There are hundreds of them in the app stores.

EATING DISORDERS:

I don't have much to say about the 1st subtype of anorexia, because I never had to deal with starving myself to such a point, but Bulimia (2nd subtype) is something that I encountered in the past.

Not only can it cause irreplaceable damage to your throat & teeth, it is often times very unrewarding. I use to overeat (binge eat). I would feel bad for eating too much. My only way out was to purge (vomit) again.

It is a vicious cycle, because after purging, my stomach would be empty. I would soon feel very hungry, eat too much again, and then purge. This cycle could continue throughout the day. I never actually lost weight. This is not something you want to play around with.

Another problem is that a lot of people overeat due to emotions. It's psychological. Pay attention to why you are over-eating. What triggers it? What did you think or feel before you ate big? Emotions that make us feel bad will often be the trigger for over eating.

If you think that you are an emotional eater and it happens constantly, then you need work on what emotions stress you out. If it is too difficult, then try therapy, meet a local dietician, or check for resources online.

WRAP UP:

Please, keep learning new things, trying new foods, read more labels, and google new ideas. I'd rather see people gaining a pound while trying, than not taking any steps at all.

I am very grateful for the weight I have lost, and it is all thanks to the information I placed in this book. I continue losing weight every year after fall hunger strikes. I want you to remember that the skinniest of people have days when they feel fat. We have good days & bad days no matter who we are, but we should love ourselves every day, no matter what we see in our reflection. With that said, I wish everyone good luck on your weight loss journey's. Thank you.

Good luck to you & thank you for reading my book. I hope everything helps.

SOURCES

1) Reviewed by Dansinger Michael, MD on (January 17, 2017) Paragraph 6. Sentence 1. *What Is Ketosis?* Retrieved from http://www.WebMD.com

2) Reviewed by Dr. Edward Group, (October 21, 2015) Paragraph 9. Sentence 4. *The Weight Loss Benefits of Hoodia Gordonii* Retrieved from https://www.globalhealingcenter.com

3) Reviewed by Lazovick Meg, (March 26, 2015) First Chart; "When Did You Wake Up This Morning?" Wake Me Up Series 2. Retrieved from http://www.edisonresearch.com

4) Reviewed by Unknown, (May 14, 2014) Third Chart; "When People Leave for Work (Excludes after 9am)" how-people-get-to-work-in-the-capital-region. Retrieved from http://alloveralbany.com

5) Reviewed by Unknown/Urban Mapping, (N/A 2011) Fifth Chart; "Time leaving home to go to work." Walmart-Distribution-Center-Bentonville-AR Retrieved from http://www.city-data.com

6) Reviewed by Waldman Katy, (JUNE 6 2012) First and Second Charts; "On Average What Time Do You Wake Up In The Morning?" & "On Average What Time Do You Go To Bed?" Do You Check Your iPhone in Bed? Retrieved from http://www.slate.com

7) Reviewed by Unknown, (N/A 2011) First Chart; "At Approximately What Time Of Day Do You Wake Up?" typical-weekday-wake-up-time-in-the-uk Retrieved from https://www.statista.com

8) Reviewed by The Pioneer Woman, (August 3, 2011) First Chart; "What Time Do You Go To Bed At Night?" photography/to-celebrate-photography Retrieved from https://thepioneerwoman.com

9) Reviewed by N/A (N/A) Understanding your Target Heart Rate Retrieved from www.active.com

10) Reviewed by National Institute of Health, (N/A) First Chart. Are-You-at-a-Healthy-Weight.pdf https://www.nhlbi.nih.gov

11) Reviewed by US Army, (N/A 2017) Whole Page Chart. US Army Male Height & Weight Standards Retrieved by http://www.apft-standards.com

12) Reviewed by US Army, (N/A 2017) Whole Page Chart. US Army Female Height & Weight Standards Retrieved by http://www.apft-standards.com

13) Reviewed by Obi Obadike, (June 13, 2012) Paragraph 2. Sentence 4. Ask The Ripped Dude: What's The Best Form Of HIIT? Retrieved by https://www.bodybuilding.com

14) Reviewed by Annalee Newitz, (May 7, 2008) Fast Food Joints Add Hormone to Food That Makes You Want to Eat More Retrieved by https://io9.gizmodo.com

15) Reviewed by N/A, (July N/A, 2016) Definition & Facts for Bariatric Surgery/ How much does bariatric surgery cost? Retrieved by https://www.niddk.nih.gov

16) Reviewed by Rita Rubin, (Jan. 16, 2015) The New Device to Treat Obesity: Is It for You? Retrieved by https://www.webmd.com

17) Reviewed by Christine Mikstas, RD, LD on (Nov 5, 2016) Paragraph 1 Sentence 1. Very Low-Calorie Diets: What You Need to Know Retrieved by https://www.webmd.com/

www.ingramcontent.com/pod-product-compliance
Lightning Source LLC
Chambersburg PA
CBHW081635250726
48657CB00009B/2896